Low Carb

The Ultimate Guide To Low Carb High Fat Diet

Practical Tips, Top Secrets, Easy-To-Follow Low Carb Recipes For Weight Loss

I0455808

Table of Contents

Introduction

Thank you for downloading this book "Low Carb: All In One Guide To Low Carb High Fat Diet."

This book contains practical tips, top secrets, and easy to follow low carb recipes for weight loss. If you want to lose weight, burn your extra fats, and stay healthy, read this book about high fat, low carb diet and it will help you achieve your weight loss goals.

Low Carb High Fat (LCHF) Diet has been making a buzz in the diet industry for quite some time now due to its numerous health benefits. LCHF diet is an effective and proven way to lose weight and keep your body healthy. If you want to be successful with it, you should know how to do it right.

This book will help you understand the basics and principles of the Low Carb High Fat Diet. In this book, you will also learn how to start the LCHF diet right and provides you with LCHF recipes that are all sumptuous and nutritious.

Don't forget to check out the bonus at the end of this book.

Thanks again for downloading this book, I hope you enjoy it!

Chapter 1 - Low Carb High Fat Diet: Basics and Principles

LCHF Diet restricts you from consuming carbohydrates that are typically found in pasta, bread, pastries and other sugary food. This diet is rich in fats, high in protein, and packed with healthy fruits and vegetables.

With this diet, you are not required to count your calories or eat and drink supplements just like other diets do. As long as you focus on eating nutritious real food that includes vegetables, natural fats and protein, you are going to be just fine.

Low carb diet means you can only consume less than 20 grams of carbohydrates each day. Your carbohydrates should come mainly from vegetables. Fiber is not restricted so you can eat more to keep you satiated.

What You Can Eat

You can eat poultry and other farm animals such as beef, lamb, chicken, pork and others. It would be best to choose grass-fed animals. If not available in your area, choose lean meat instead.

Any kind of fish is allowed but of course, fresh, wild-caught fish is best. Mussels, crabs, lobsters, other shells and clams are also allowed. Pastured eggs, cheese, heavy cream, yogurt, and butter are also accepted.

Fresh, organic vegetables are recommended but if it is not possible, you can opt for packed or dried as long as they do not contain preservatives and are not processed.

Since some fruits contain more sugar than others, limit them to oranges, strawberries, apples, blueberries, and pears. You can also have some seeds and nuts such as sunflower seeds, walnuts, and almonds among others.

Unlike other diets that restrict saturated fats, the low-carb diet encourages you to consume them. You can make use of coconut oil, olive oil, lard, almond oil, and cod fish liver oil.

If your goal is to lose weight, you have to refrain from eating tuber, non-gluten grains, legumes, dark chocolates, and wine. But, if you are active and your goal is to stay healthy, you can afford to be a bit lax with potatoes, sweet potatoes, and other tubers. You can also have some oats, quinoa, rice, and other grains. If you can tolerate legumes, you may also have some black beans, pinto beans, lentils and others. You can also have some dark chocolate as long as it is 70% cocoa or higher. You can also have a glass of wine as long as it has no added sugars and carbs.

Dark chocolate is an antioxidant that can provide health benefits if consumed in moderation. Wine is also known to boost heart health when taken in moderation. Please be reminded that chocolate and wine can prevent/hinder your progress if you consume too much of them.

Keep yourself hydrated at all times. Water is an antioxidant and it helps cleanse your body of unwanted toxins. You can also drink tea and coffee as long as in moderation.

What You Cannot Eat

Low carb diet only restricts food that are not good for you. Candy, ice cream, fruit juices, soft drinks, agave, and other products that contain refined sugars are not allowed. Refined sugars are empty calories that make you feel hungry and crave for more sugar-laden food.

Grains that are rich in gluten are also not allowed. These grains can cause gluten intolerance that can lead to autoimmune diseases. Wheat, barley, rye, and spelt are high-gluten grains. Breads, pasta, and any product that contains these grains are also not allowed.

You can eat any type of fruit, but you should limit them to 1 cup only. If you are diabetic, limit your fruit intake to ½ cup only. Large fruits contain more carbs and you have to watch your carb intake as it can influence your blood sugar more than any other nutrients. Although oranges, apples, and pears have less carbs, they do come in large sizes. Choose the smallest size as one large apple contains 30g of carbohydrates. Same goes with other crunchy fruits such as pears, persimmon, and oranges.

Dried fruits must be avoided if you have Type 2 Diabetes. Since they are dehydrated, you tend to eat more and it is easy to overeat. If you really want to eat some, keep it to 1 to 2 tablespoons only. If you eat ½ cup of dried berries, figs, banana, apples or raisins, they can add up to 50g to 60g of carbohydrates.

Fruit juices usually lack fiber, making them less satisfying. If you are healthy, one cup will not hurt. But, if you are Diabetic, you have to keep your consumption to 4 ounces as it can result to a quick rise in your blood sugar levels. Consuming 12 oz to 16 oz of fruit juice contains 40-50 grams of carbohydrates.

Trans Fats are fats found in processed food and oils. Refrain from using hydrogenated oils, partially hydrogenated oils, and refined oils as they went through heavy chemical processing. Trans Fats are not easily digested by your body and are stored as fats in your cells, which slow down your metabolism. Vegetable oils and seed oils such as soybean oil, safflower oil, corn oil, sunflower oil, canola oil, and grape seed oil are also not allowed as they are not easily digested by your body.

Refined sugar and other artificial sweeteners are not allowed. They are calorie-filled and can cause quick blood spikes with those who are suffering from diabetes. Watch out for food or drinks that contain aspartame, cyclamates, saccharin, sucralose, acesulfame potassium and other artificial sweeteners. If you want to sweeten your dishes, you can use Stevia, honey or maple syrup instead but in moderation.

Stay away from low fat, diet, and processed food. The natural composition of these food have been altered and have gone through heavy processing. Make sure to read the label of the products you buy. If they contain more than 3 ingredients, they are either preserved or processed, even when if they are labeled as "healthy food".

Chapter 2   Tips on How to Do the Low Carb High Fat Diet the Right Way

Low Carb Diet is quite simple, you just have to ditch the bad stuff and take in the good ones. Everything must be in moderation. You know your body. When you are full, stop eating. Eat when you are hungry.

To start, don't jump ahead. Take it little by little. Every step you make is important and there is no need to hurry. Start by eating less processed food and replace them with vegetables that you enjoy the most. Incorporate fruits and vegetables on your meals by making a smoothie. Instead of bingeing on chips, eat a palmful of nuts instead.

Give yourself a week. Slowly incorporate fruits, vegetables, and lean meat to your meals. Slowly get rid of processed food and junk food in your refrigerator. If you are addicted to sweets, instead of eating 2 cupcakes a day, reduce it to once a day then completely eliminate them from your system.

Do the same with alcohol and smoke. Going cold turkey is not the right way. Slowly reduce your consumption day by day. After a week, you should be ready for the LCHF diet.

Even when you are in a low-carb diet, you can still enjoy eating at restaurants and attending parties with your friends. Choose dishes that are meat-based or fish-based. If the food is fried, ask them to fry it in butter or lard. Instead of bread and pasta, ask for vegetables instead.

When you go shopping, go straight to the fresh produce section. Although organic is best, you can still go for fresh, whole food offered in grocery stores. Dried vegetables can be alternatives as long as they are not processed and they do not contain preservatives. You can also use canned fruits and vegetables, but you have to read the labels carefully.

Shopping Tips:

Make a list of your desired recipes for the week. Organize the ingredients from least to many so that you can distinguish which ones to buy in bulk. It is better to store your spices as they have long shelf life provided you store them properly.

Do your groceries in a weekly basis. Fruits and vegetables are perishable so you have to store them properly. To prolong their shelf life, you can pre cut them, store them in sealed containers or resealable bags and store them in the freezer.

You can save more time and money if you cook your food beforehand. Since you already have your recipes planned for the week, cook them during the weekends and store them in the freezer. All you have to do is heat them when needed. Don't forget to label the containers as you need to know which to consume first to prevent wasting food.

Sample Menu for A Week

This sample menu provides less than 50 grams of total carbohydrates per day. If you are not trying to lose weight and you just want to keep your body healthy, you can go a bit lax and have more than 50 grams of carbs per day, but do not exceed 80 grams.

Monday

Breakfast: Egg omelet with mushrooms, sautéed in coconut oil, butter or lard.

Lunch: Lean pork steak with vegetables

Dinner: Chicken marinade with freshly squeezed orange juice

Tuesday

Breakfast: Yogurt with ½ cup blueberries and a palmful of almonds

Lunch: Cheeseburger without buns, salsa and vegetables

Dinner: Grilled salmon with vegetables

Wednesday

Breakfast: Leftover veggies and salmon from last night

Lunch: Chicken salad with green veggies

Dinner: Shrimp cooked in butter

Thursday

Breakfast: Fried egg with vegetables on the side

Lunch: Any leftover from previous days

Dinner: Beef with broccoli or asparagus

Friday

Breakfast: Beaten egg with bacon bits

Lunch: Citrus salad with steamed chicken strips

Dinner: Beef patties with vegetables

Saturday

Breakfast: Bacon and eggs

Lunch: Any leftovers from the day before with a cup of mixed fruits

Dinner: Chicken marinade with vegetables on the side

Sunday

Breakfast: Blueberry smoothie with coconut milk

Lunch: Pork chops in coconut oil with veggies

Dinner: Grilled salmon with salsa and veggies

You can be more flexible with your recipes as long as they have more low-carb vegetables. If you are trying to lose weight, limit your fruit intake to one per day and splurge on leafy greens and low-carb veggies. If you are active and you just want to maintain your health, you can add sweet potatoes, potatoes, rice and oats to your diet, but keep them to a minimum.

Chapter 3   The Secret To LCHF Diet

The effect of LCHF Diet to an individual varies. Some may experience side effects but some may not. To minimize these side effects, you should do the transition gradually. Plan when you will start with the diet. Before you do so, you have to prepare your kitchen. Make sure everything you have in your kitchen is according to the principles of this diet.

How to Minimize Side Effects

If you experience any of the symptoms enumerated below, follow the guidelines to minimize and relieve their effects.

Induction Flu – These are flu-like symptoms that include headache, nausea, lethargy, irritability, confusion, and brain fog. They are commonly experienced in your first 2 to 4 days. Usually, you will feel unmotivated, tired, and lethargic. These symptoms typically go away by themselves, but you can also prevent them from happening. All you need is more water and add some salt in your diet.

If you experience these symptoms, try mixing a glass of water with ½ teaspoon salt. Drink it and your symptoms will usually go away after 15 to 30 minutes. Increase your water intake to keep your body hydrated.

Tip:

Do not starve yourself. Add more fats to your diet to keep you satiated and energetic. You have a lot of options, but if in doubt, add more coconut oil or butter to your dishes.

If your symptoms don't go away after 3 days, you can increase your carb intake but keep it to 50 grams per day and not exceeding 80 grams. This is not ideal as your transition will be slower, but it will help your body adjust better to the change in your diet.

Leg Cramps – Some individuals may experience leg cramps during the transition. If this happens to you, drink a glass of water with ½ teaspoon salt. If necessary, you may take slow release magnesium supplements. If the symptoms still persist, add your carbohydrates intake however, this will reduce the effects of the low carb diet.

Constipation – Since your body is not well adapted to a low-carb diet, you may experience constipation. Drink at least 12 glasses of water each day and add some extra salt. Increase your vegetable intake as they are full of fiber, which supports better bowel movement. Choose non-starchy vegetables and focus more on leafy greens to help solve this issue.

Bad Breath – This may not be the case for all but you may experience it especially on the first two weeks of your diet. For some, this condition is just temporary and goes away after a week or two after the body has well adjusted to the diet. Bad breath happens as a result of ketosis. Your body burns more fats, which are converted to ketones, an acetone that fuels the brain. In some cases, ketones turn up as bad breath or body odor when you are working out and sweating too much. What you can do is drink more water especially when your mouth is drying. This is an indication that your body is dehydrating and you don't have enough saliva to flush away bacteria in your mouth. Add a little salt in your diet, too.

Remember to brush at least twice a day to minimize the odor. You may also use mouthwash to mask the smell. If the smell does not go away after two weeks, eat more carbohydrates. You can eat 50 to 70 grams of carbohydrates a day but do not go beyond 80 grams. Doing so can reduce the weight loss effects of the low carb diet.

Another option is to go intermittent with the low carb diet. You can have 20 grams or lower carbohydrates for your first 3 days and consume 50 to 70 grams of carbohydrates for the next two days.

Heart Palpitations – This is a common symptom during the first week of going through the low carb diet. Dehydration and lack of salt cause your heart to pump a bit harder to maintain proper blood pressure. You can cure this symptom by drinking more water and making sure you get enough salt. If your heart palpitations do not stop, add your carb intake to 50 to 70 grams per day. You can gradually decrease your carb intake after your heart palpitations are relieved.

If you are diabetic, you need to test your blood sugar level from time to time as low carb diet can result to low blood sugar or high blood pressure, which can result to heart palpitations. If this happens, consult your doctor as you may need to reduce your medication.

Lowered Physical Performance – This is a typical symptom since your body is adapting to the diet. Your body is not used to burning fats for energy and it takes a few weeks or even months for the body to adapt. Your physical performance will improve faster when you exercise while on a diet.

Going on a low carb diet reduces your body fat, which results to lightening of your body. This will increase your physical abilities as you are able to move freely with an increased energy.

In general, the side effects of LCHF diet can be relieved by drinking more water and adding more salt to your diet. If this solution does not work, it means your body cannot tolerate low carbs so you have to consume more. This will reduce the benefits of low carb diet when it comes to weight loss. Gradually, your body will be able to adapt and you can reduce your carb consumption to 20 grams daily for maximum effect.

Chapter 4   Health Benefits Of Low Carb Diet

The LCHF Diet is getting a lot of attention from the health community because of its numerous health benefits. The LCHF diet helps lower insulin and glucose levels. Excess glucose gets stored in your body as fats. Additionally, high insulin level results to Diabetes which compromises your immunity and metabolism.

The LCHF diet allows you to consume more saturated fats from cheese and red meat. According to studies, LCHF diet results to weight loss and reduces the risk of heart diseases similar to Atkins Diet, Zone Diet, and Weight Watchers Plan.

Going on a low carb diet also helps keep your blood pressure to normal. High blood pressure increases your risk of having heart attack and stroke. The Western Diet is laced with sugar, salt, and lots of carbohydrates. When you go low carb, you get rid of unhealthy food that cause elevated blood pressure, making you healthier and more aware of the food that you eat.

Another great benefit of going low carb is reduced acne. This is no coincidence. Many people have experienced improvements in their acne after going through the LCHF diet. Experts believed that this has to do with insulin levels and growth hormones such as IGF. To improve acne, dairy-free low carb diet is recommended.

Low carb diet also provides therapeutic effects on people with epilepsy. Since the 1920's, the low carb diet is already used to control symptoms of children with epilepsy. Many studies prove that low carb diet decreases the incident of seizures in patients who are suffering from epilepsy. In some cases, adults with epilepsy who are in a low carb diet are able to take lesser medications. Some are able to go seizure-free without medication.

ADHD symptoms can also be reduced with LCHF diet. Although this claim is yet to be proven by science, many parents have experienced a reduction of symptoms in their kids who have ADHD as well as in adults who have the same condition. It is believed that the elimination of junk food and the reduction of sugar and carbohydrates intake help reduce the symptoms.

Going on a low carb diet means you will eat more healthy vegetables and get rid of highly processed food and carbohydrates. Vegetables are antioxidants and they contain nutrients that keep your skin, hair, and nails healthy. They are also filled with fiber that supports better digestion and nutrient absorption.

Going on a low carb diet is not only for those who wish to lose weight. It is also for those people who want to be healthier and control their symptoms.

Chapter 5　Low Carb Recipes You Can Enjoy

These low-carb recipes are so delicious; you will forget you are on a diet. They are fulfilling and satisfying and they are easy to prepare. You can prepare these dishes for your family and friends in various occasions.

Grain –Free Breakfast Granola

Ingredients:

150 grams	Sunflower Seeds
150 grams	Dried Fennel Seeds
150 grams	Pumpkin Seeds
2 tablespoons	Ground Cardamom
2 tablespoons	Ground Ginger
400 grams unsweetened	Shredded/Desiccated Coconut,
150 grams	Coconut Oil, melted
4 to 6 tablespoons	Stevia, honey or maple syrup

Directions:

1. Preheat your oven to 350°F.

2. In a large roasting dish, mix all ingredients together.

3. Roast for 20 minutes, turning the mixture every 3 to 4 minutes. Set your timer to prevent the mixture from burning.

4. When all the ingredients are brown and evenly roasted, remove from oven and cool completely.

5. Store in mason jars or glass containers with tight lid. It can last up to a week in the refrigerator.

Low Carb Meatloaf

Ingredients:

1.5 lbs	Ground lean beef/pork/turkey or any meat of your choice
2 large	Eggs, beaten
1 large	Red Onion, diced
1 pinch	Salt
1 pinch	Ground Black Pepper
100 grams	Grated Parmesan Cheese
2 slices	Bacon, diced
1 handful	Fresh Basil, chopped
1 handful	Fresh Parsley, chopped
¼ cup	Sundried Tomatoes, diced
2 teaspoons	Dried Oregano

Directions:

1. In a large bowl, mix together ground meat, onions, salt, pepper and egg.

2. Stir in bacon, basil, parsley, tomatoes and oregano.

3. Preheat you oven to 350°F.

4. Slightly oil your muffin tray and set aside.

5. Scoop out the mix mixture with spoon and place them in each of the muffin holes. Press the mixture down but not too hard.

6. Top with grated parmesan cheese.

7. Bake until all sides are brown and the cheese has melted.

Wheat-Free Coconut Pancake

Ingredients:

150 grams	Desiccated Coconut
½ cup	Coconut Flour
1 cup	Coconut Cream
4	Eggs
4	Ripe Bananas, mashed
3 teaspoons	Stevia, honey or maple syrup
1 teaspoon	Ground Cinnamon
1 teaspoon	Vanilla Paste
2 teaspoons	Baking Powder
2 tablespoons	Butter

Directions:

1. In a large mixing bowl, combine mashed bananas and eggs. Add one egg at a time while mixing.

2. Stir in coconut cream. Mix until fully incorporated.

3. Add the rest of the ingredients. Use a stick blender for a smooth batter.

4. Heat your non-stick pan over medium heat and melt the butter.

5. Place a spoonful of the mixture in the pan and fry until golden brown on both sides. Make sure to brown the pan cake before flipping to the other side.

6. If necessary, add more coconut flour to make the batter firm.

Smoked Salmon In Scrambled Eggs

Ingredients:

1 oz	Butter
2 cups	Baby Spinach, chopped roughly
2	Eggs
2 tablespoons	Full Fat Cream
2 oz	Smoked Salmon
1 oz	Full Fat Cream Cheese
1 pinch	Salt
1 pinch	Ground Black Pepper

1. Heat your frying pan over medium heat and melt half of the butter.

2. Sauté spinach and season with salt and pepper. Cook until leafy greens are wilted. Transfer in a serving plate and set aside.

3. In a bowl. Whisk together milk and eggs until fully incorporated.

4. Melt the rest of the butter in the frying pan. Add the egg mixture and stir gently to make the scrambled eggs fluffy.

5. Place the smoked salmon on top of the greens. Top with warm scrambled eggs and garnish with cream cheese.

Chocó Berry Green Smoothie

Ingredients:

½ cup	Frozen Berries of your choice
100 grams	Baby Spinach, stemmed
1 cup	Coconut Cream
¼ cup	Cocoa Powder
1 tablespoon	Granulated Stevia/Honey/Maple Syrup

Directions:

1. Place all ingredients in your blender and whiz until smooth.

2. Blend it until the spinach leaves are no longer noticeable to make it more appealing to children.

Citrus Chicken With Rosemary

Ingredients:

5 pieces fillet)	Chicken (breasts, thigh, legs or
1 small	Lemon, juice and zest
3 tablespoons	Olive Oil /Coconut Oil
2 teaspoons	Dried Rosemary
2 cloves	Garlic, crushed and minced
1 pinch	Salt
1 pinch	Ground Black Pepper

Directions:

1. Preheat your oven to 350°F.

2. In a baking dish, mix together your choice of oil, lemon zest, lemon juice, rosemary, salt and pepper.

3. Add the chicken and mix to coat every piece evenly.

4. Roast for 30 minutes while occasionally basting the chicken with its juices.

Salmon Veggie Sushi

Ingredients:

1 sticks	Carrot, peeled and sliced into ½ inch long
1 unpeeled	Cucumber, cut into ½ inch long strips,
½ lb strips	Smoked Salmon, cut into ½ inch long
1 cup needed	Full Fat Cream Cheese, add more if

Directions:

1. In a bowl, soften the cream cheese by mixing it with fork.

2. Add the salmon strips and mix.

3. Place a large nori sheet on your working space. Add the salmon-cream cheese mixture on one side and leave a 1-inch strip on the other side of the nori.

4. Add the vegetable strips on the center of the cream cheese-salmon mix. Wet the left space on the other side of the nori with water. Roll the nori and lock it on the wet strip.

5. When done, cut the nori rolls into smaller pieces and refrigerate.

Chicken Tandoori Bites

Ingredients:

2 large pieces	Chicken Breasts cut into 8 smaller
¼ cup	Yogurt or Geek, unsweetened
2 tablespoons	Tandoori Paste, unsweetened

Directions:

1. Mix tandoori paste and yoghurt in a bowl.

2. Mix in chicken breasts and make sure everything is evenly coated. Marinate for 2 to 4 hours in the refrigerator.

3. You can choose to barbecue, roast, and bake or fry the chicken marinade.

4. Serve with vegetables on the side.

Chicken Burger

Ingredients:

For the chicken burger

500 grams	Chicken, deboned and minced
1 large	Red onion, minced finely (divided)
½ teaspoon	Dried Chili
1 teaspoon	Paprika
1 clove	Garlic, crushed and minced
1 tablespoon	Cumin Powder
1 tablespoon	Dried Coriander
1 large	Egg, beaten slightly
1 cup	Coconut Oil/Olive Oil

For the avocado salsa

1 teaspoon	Capsicum
1 large	Tomato, cut into small cubes
1 medium	Avocado, peeled, seeded and cut into small cubes
2 tablespoons	Cream Cheese
1 teaspoon	Chili Flakes

Directions:

1. In a mixing bowl, mix together all the ingredients for chicken burger except for the oil.

2. Heat a medium deep pot in the stove over medium heat.

3. Meanwhile, combine all the ingredients for avocado salsa in a separate bowl. Toss to coat evenly.

4. Add oil in the heated pan. Spoon the chicken mixture and shape into burger patties.

5. Fry the chicken patties until golden brown and cooked through and through.

6. Top with avocado salsa. Use thin tomato slices as buns.

Meatloaf Overload

Ingredients:

750 grams	Ground Beef
750 grams	Ground Pork
1	Spring Onion, sliced
2 cloves	Garlic, crushed and minced
1 handful	Fresh Parsley, chopped
1 handful	Fresh Basil, chopped
2 large	Eggs, beaten slightly
2 slices	Bacon, diced
14 slices	Bacon (add more if needed)
30 grams	Sun-dried Tomatoes, chopped
2 teaspoons	Dried Oregano
¼ teaspoon	Salt
¼ teaspoon	Ground Black Pepper
100 grams	Parmesan Cheese, grated

Directions:

1. Preheat your oven at 350°F.
2. Slightly oil your baking tray and set aside.
3. In a large mixing bowl, mix all the ingredients together until well blended.

4. Shape mixture into meatloaf and place on the oiled baking tray.

5. Top the meatloaf with bacon slices until fully covered.

6. Sprinkle with grated parmesan cheese.

7. Bake for 50 to 55 minutes or until fully cooked in the middle.

Pepperoni Balls

Ingredients:

500 grams	Ground Beef/Pork/Turkey
100 grams	Pepperoni, diced finely
1 pinch	Salt
1 pinch	Pepper

Directions:

1. Mix all the ingredients together.

2. Preheat your oven to 350°F.

3. Spoon some of the mixture and squeeze with your hands to bind the meat together. Do this while forming the meat mixture into a ball.

4. Oil your baking tray and arrange the meat balls for baking.

5. Bake for 15 to 20 minutes or until golden brown.

6. Turn the meatballs at least once to ensure all sides of the meatballs are evenly cooked.

Low Carb Caesar Salad

Ingredients:

1 handful	Baby Kale
1	Spring Onion, sliced
4	Cherry Tomatoes cut into halves
1 small	Cucumber, cut into cubes
1 small	Chicken Breast, steamed and pulled
2 tablespoons	Blue Cheese
½ cup	Grated Parmesan Cheese
2 tablespoons	Homemade Mayonnaise
1 tablespoon	Anchovies

Directions:

1. In a salad bowl, layer the baby kale leaves in the bottom.

2. Arrange chicken on top of the leaves. Add the cheeses.

3. Top with anchovies.

4. Add cherry tomatoes, onions and cucumbers.

5. Drizzle with homemade mayonnaise.

Pizza Waffles

Ingredients:

4 tablespoons	Coconut Flour
5 medium	Eggs, separated
1 tablespoon	Dried Rosemary
1 tablespoon	Dried Oregano
1 tablespoon	Dried Basil
1 pinch	Salt
1 pinch	Ground Black Pepper
1 teaspoon	Baking Powder
3 tablespoons	Full Fat Milk
1 stick	Butter, melted
1 tablespoon	Butter, additional
½ cup grated	Parmesan/Mozzarella Cheese,

Directions:

1. In a bowl, whisk the egg whites until stiff peaks are formed.

2. In a separate bowl, mix together egg yolks, salt, pepper, dried herbs, coconut flour and baking soda.

3. Gradually add melted butter while mixing to ensure smooth consistency.

4. Stir in grated cheese and milk.

5. Fold the egg white mixture gently into the batter until fully incorporated.

6. Oil the waffle maker with melted butter. Spoon batter into the waffle maker and cook until golden.

7. Repeat process until all batter is used up.

8. Top with your favorite toppings.

Coconut Fish Curry

Ingredients:

1kg	Fish Fillet, your choice, cut into cubes
4 tablespoons	Curry Paste
400 ml	Coconut Cream
400 ml	Water
500 grams	Spinach, washed, drained and sliced
1 tablespoon	Coconut Oil

Directions:

1. Heat coconut oil in a large saucepan. Sauté curry paste until aromatic and activated.

2. Mix in coconut cream and water. Bring to a boil.

3. Lower down heat and add fish cubes. Simmer until fish cubes are fully cooked.

4. Add spinach leaves and cook until wilted.

5. Serve while hot.

6	Chicken Drumsticks
1 cup	Almond Meal
½ teaspoon	Ginger Powder
½ teaspoon	Dried Parsley
1 teaspoon	Paprika
¼ teaspoon	Chili Powder
½ teaspoon	Dried Sage
½ teaspoon	Mustard Powder
¼ teaspoon	Five Spice
½ teaspoon	Dried Basil
1 pinch	Salt
1 pinch	Ground Black Pepper
1 cup	Lard/Coconut Oil, add more if needed

Directions:

1. In a plastic bag or resealable bag, put together almond meal and all the herbs and spices. Close/twist the top and shake vigorously to mix.

2. Add the chicken drumsticks, shake and rub the mixture into the chicken.

3. In a deep pot, heat coconut oil/lard over medium heat. Add more oil if needed. Chicken must be well covered for even frying.

4. Fry chicken until golden brown or cooked through and through.

5. Drain excess oil and serve.

These recipes are all low-carb, easy to prepare and tasty. You can prepare them for your friends and family for all occasions. Your kids will surely enjoy them without second thoughts.

Check out the bonus recipes below:

BONUS!!!

Low Carb Slow Cooker Recipes For Weight Loss

Slow Cooker Bacon and Pumpkin Soup

Ingredients:

1	Bacon Hock (pig joint)
2 lbs	Pumpkin, diced
2 to 3 cups	Boiling Water
1 pinch	Salt
1 pinch	Pepper

Directions:

1. Place the bacon hock and pumpkin in the slow cooker.

2. Add boiling water. Make sure the ingredients are covered with water.

3. Cook on high for 3 to 4 hours or 6 to 10 on low.

4. When you see the meat falling off from the bones, remove carefully and place on the chopping board.

5. Pull the meat from the bone. Discard the bone and put the meat back into the slow cooker.

6. When done, puree with stick blender until smooth.

7. Serve with cream cheese or sour cream. You may top with chopped basil if you want.

Slow Cooker Meatballs

Ingredients:

1kg	Ground Beef
1 large	Onion, quartered
2 slices	Bacon, diced
2 cloves	Garlic, peeled
1 teaspoon	Dried Rosemary
1 teaspoon	Thyme
1 teaspoon	Oregano
1 teaspoon	Marjoram
1 teaspoon	Sage
1 large	Egg, beaten slightly
1 pinch	Salt
1 pinch	Pepper
2 cups	Tomatoes, chopped

Directions:

1. Oil the bottom and sides of your slow cooker.

2. In a blender or food processor, pulse together garlic, bacon and onion until chopped finely.

3. Add ground beef, egg, herbs and spices. Pulse until smooth.

4. Transfer in a bowl and form mixture into meat balls.

5. Place meatballs in the slow cooker.

6. Add chopped tomatoes. Season with salt and pepper.

7. Cook in low for 6 to 10 hours or on high for 4 to 6 hours depending on your slow cooker.

Slow Cooker Chicken Marinade

Ingredients:

1kg	Chicken, all parts
3 tablespoons	Apple Cider Vinegar
2 tablespoons	Soy Sauce
1 teaspoon	Black Pepper, whole
1 large	Red Onion, sliced
5 cloves	Garlic, crushed
4 leaves	Dried Laurel
1 pinch	Salt
1 pinch	Ground Black Pepper
¼ cup	Water

Directions:

1. Mix vinegar, soy sauce and water in the slow cooker.

2. Add chicken, herbs and spices.

3. Mix until all chicken parts are covered with sauce.

4. Cook in low for 4 to 5 hours or on high for 6 to 8 hours depending on your slow cooker.

Slow Cooker Beef Curry

Ingredients:

800 grams	Beef, cut into small pieces
1 cup	Coconut Cream
1 large	Red Onion, quartered
1 teaspoon	Ground Cardamom
1 teaspoon	Five Spice
1 teaspoon	Ground Cinnamon
1 teaspoon	Turmeric Powder
1 teaspoon	Ground Cumin
½ teaspoon	Chili Powder
2 teaspoons	Ground Coriander
4	Cloves
1 handful	Spinach, stemmed

Directions:

1. Put all ingredients in the slow cooker except the spinach.

2. Mix all ingredients until all beef slices are evenly covered with sauce.

3. Cook on low for 8 to 10 hours or on high for 4 to 6 hours.

4. Before serving, add the spinach and cook for 5 more minutes.

Slow Cooker Poached Citrus Salmon

Ingredients:

4 to 6	Salmon Fillets, skin-on
2 cups	Water
1 cup	Dry White Wine
6 sprigs	Fresh Dill
1 fruit	Lemon, sliced thinly
1 fruit	Lemon, cut into wedges
1	Shallot, sliced thinly
1	Bay Leaf
1 teaspoon	Salt
1 teaspoon	Black Pepper, whole
2 tablespoons	Olive Oil

Directions:

1. In your slow cooker, mix together water, wine, bay leaf, black pepper, shallots, dill and salt.

2. Season top of salmon with salt and pepper and place in the slow cooker. Cook for 45 minutes on low or until the meat starts to flake with fork.

3. When done, drizzle with olive oil and sprinkle with salt. Serve with lemon wedges and leafy greens on the side.

Slow cooker comes in handy specially when you are busy and not have enough time to cook. You just place all the ingredients in your slow cooker and let it do the cooking. You can go about your daily tasks while cooking your meal. You can prepare your slow cooker recipes at night and wake up to a delicious breakfast in the morning.

You can cook your food in batches and store them properly in the freezer so you can just reheat when needed.

Conclusion

Thank you again for downloading this book!

I hope this book was able to help you to understand the Low Carb High Fat Diet and use it to achieve your desired body. The LCHF diet is not only for weight loss, it also keeps your body healthy and helps relieve symptoms of various diseases and conditions.

Remember, you do not need to starve yourself when you go on a diet. It is not true that fats are bad. Saturated fats are good for your health and they do not make you fat. The principle of LCHF diet is simple: minimize your starches, stay away from processed foods, no to refined sugars and refined oils and eat more nutritious, real foods such as fruits, vegetables, fish and meat.

As with everything else, take one step at a time. Do not aim for fast results. Instead, aim for long-term results. You will not be able to experience the full benefits of the LCHF diet if you take shortcuts. You will just rebound back to where you started off. You must focus on your objective and be happy with your results no matter how small they are.

If you enjoyed this book, then I'd like to ask you for a favor, would you be kind enough to leave a review for this book on Amazon? It'd be greatly appreciated!

Thank you and good luck!

www.ingramcontent.com/pod-product-compliance
Lightning Source LLC
Chambersburg PA
CBHW072018290526
45787CB00013B/1299